DIY Homemade Medical Face Mask: How to Make Your Own Medical Face Mask for Protection Against Bacteria, Viruses, and Disease

Kenneth Olsen

Table of Contents

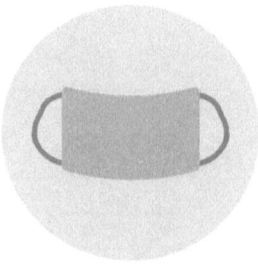

Introduction

We live in uncertain times. While humanity has made huge leaps in medicine and our understanding of diseases, we're still very vulnerable. Even in developed countries, diseases can spread quickly with devastating consequences. How do we protect ourselves? We can't just rely on our governments to protect us. We have to control the things we have control over and do what we can to stay safe.

In this book, I'll discuss how to make homemade face masks. These are a common sight these days. Most importantly, I'll also talk about what masks can and can't do for your health. Knowing how and when to wear a mask and what else you need to do to protect your health could save lives. You'll learn the differences between face masks and respirators, how to sew your own mask, and how to take care of your mask. With this information, you can protect yourself, your family, and your community.

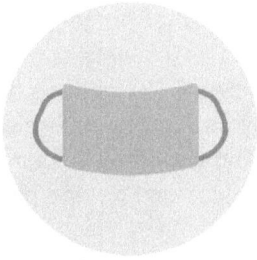

Chapter 1: The History of Medical Masks

When did humans figure out that masks could protect them from certain diseases? We had some idea that it could be helpful, but before germ theory, our understanding of what caused disease was off. It took many years of development to get the masks we have today. In this chapter, you'll learn about the history of medical masks, the different types, and why masks become such a hot commodity during disease outbreaks.

Two main types of masks

There are two main types of medical masks: surgical masks and respirators. Surgical masks (also known generally as "face masks") have a loose fit. Healthcare workers and caregivers use these most of the time. The masks block large droplets created by sneezing and coughing, protecting patients from bacteria. People in the general public (who are ill) also wear masks to prevent spreading the droplets.

Respirators (N95 respirators are the best known) fit more tightly. N95 respirators are used in both the medical and industrial fields. They block 95% of airborne particles and are able to block smaller particles than regular face masks. While surgical masks don't prevent healthy people from inhaling particles, N95 respirators do. Because N95 respirators are tricky to fit, authorities don't recommend them for the general public. If worn incorrectly, they aren't effective.

The first masks

The most iconic image of a face mask from the past has got to be the bird-like masks from the Black Plague. During this time, doctors had no idea what germs were or what was causing the plague. In fact, since the bubonic plague was actually spread by fleas carried around on rats, face masks wouldn't help!

Even if it had been spread through the air, people weren't covering their faces to block droplets. Everyone believed that bad-smelling gases from the ground caused the disease. Known as "miasma," these gases were supposedly created by rotting organic matter and lead to every kind of disease like cholera and the plague. Those terrifying bird masks weren't for show. They had two nostril holes at the end, so the beaks could be stuffed with incense. The thinking was if the doctor could block the miasma with something that smelled good, they wouldn't get the plague.

For everyone who didn't have one of these fancy masks, they covered their faces with their sleeves or handkerchiefs. According to folklore, a group of thieves who robbed the dead made a mixture of spices, rubbed it on cloth, and tied it over their mouths and noses. That's the story of *Thieves Essential Oil*, which you may hear a lot about during flu season and disease outbreaks. We're not going to talk about essential oil in this book, but it's an interesting fact from the same time as early face masks.

Surgical masks

Doctors started wearing the first surgical masks in the late 19th century. A French surgeon, Paul Berger, used it during an operation. These masks weren't intended to filter out particles from airborne diseases, but rather to prevent the doctor from getting their droplets into a patient's open surgical wounds. Soon, all doctors and then other members of the health field began using masks, so they weren't just for surgeries anymore. However, the mask's intent is still not to protect the person wearing the mask, but everyone else. They aren't designed to protect you from bacteria or viruses, but if you're sick, the masks block your droplets. If there's a filter material in the mask, this can prevent some inhalation of particles, but they're not considered reliable.

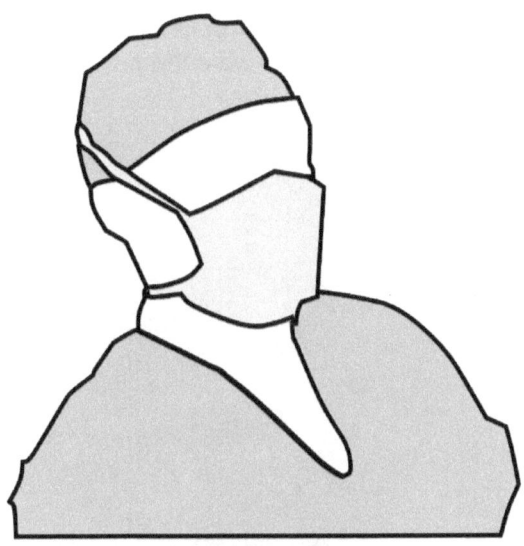

Loose fit on face.
Meant for sick people, medical staff, and people caring for sick people.
Does not prevent inhalation of particles.

It's very common to see people wearing surgical masks in East Asian countries, especially during flu season. The air quality is notoriously poor, so many believe people wear masks for that reason, but regular surgical masks aren't effective against pollution. Some help a little - if they're worn correctly and made of thick material - but most don't do anything. Because masks are so prevalent in East Asia, many companies release fashionable masks.

The respirator mask

The type of mask you'll hear about a lot these days is the N95 mask. This is a type of respirator, which as we mentioned earlier, has a tight fit and can actually block virus particles. It's also effective against air pollution. What's the story behind this mask?

In 1910, a horrific plague spread across Northern China. With a mortality rate of 100%, it ended up killing between 50,000-60,000 people. It was a pneumonic plague, which includes symptoms like fever, headache, and pneumonia that develops very quickly. To deal with this disease, a doctor named Wu Lien-teh was brought in. He figured out that the plague was airborne. Having seen masks used in the Western world, Wu designed his own mask made from more durable cotton and gauze. He added several cloth layers. Despite some early doubts, people saw that Wu's mask worked. Best of all, the mask was easy and cheap to make. Countless masks went into production. Soon, everyone from doctors to soldiers to civilians wore them.

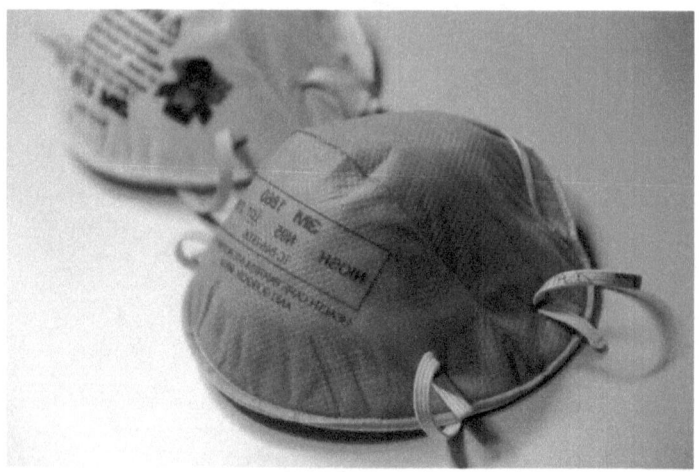

Fits tightly on face.
Designed to block inhalation of particles.
Used in industrial and medical fields.

Over time, people and companies kept improving on Wu's design. Eventually, we ended up with the N95 mask. They were actually mainly used for industrial purposes. Materials like fiberglass filters were added. 3M designed the first single-use N95 respirator in the early 1970s. It wasn't until the 1990s when drug-resistant tuberculosis became a huge problem. Healthcare workers were at risk of catching the disease when caring for patients. To provide protective equipment, the standards for the N95 respirator were tweaked for the health field.

While essential for medical workers, N95 respirators are not used that often. That's why when they are required, it's a really big deal. Most of the time, regular masks are sufficient. N95 respirators are still used in the industrial field on a frequent basis.

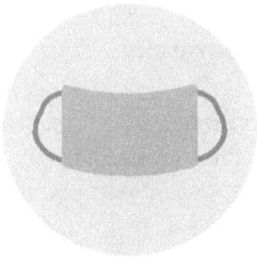

Chapter 2: When Do I Need To Use A Mask?

You know a bit about the history of masks and what they're used for. How do you know when you should wear one? In this chapter, we'll talk about the types of diseases a mask can defend against, the pros and cons of a mask, and when you should consider wearing one.

Diseases

Surgical masks, when worn properly, can protect a community against diseases that spread by droplets. Droplet-spread diseases include the common cold, the flu, rubella, and viruses. A study from 2013 showed that surgical masks reduced the amount of virus spray by three times. This means that the person who was sick wore the mask. I want to be clear that regular surgical masks are not designed to protect healthy people from getting sick, but they are better than nothing. We'll get into why it's still worthwhile to learn how to make your own mask a bit later on.

Diseases don't only spread by droplets. Some infections spread when a person who is sick talks, breathes, sneezes, or coughs. These actions release tiny particles called small particle aerosols. Because they are so small, they can travel long distances with the wind and live in the air as long as hours. This is what people mean when they say a disease is "airborne." Others can breathe in these particles and get sick, even if they weren't in direct contact with the original ill person. These types of diseases include measles, tuberculosis, and chickenpox. Because these virus particles are so small, an N95 respirator is the only dependable mask that filters out the disease.

Pros and cons of homemade masks

Homemade masks become more common during disease outbreaks. The masks and respirators that aren't collected by the medical community are quickly bought up by the general public. Prices can go up, as well. When you don't have other options, what are the pros and cons of homemade masks?

Pro: Wearing a homemade mask is better than nothing

Data shows that when sick people wear homemade masks, the masks aren't as effective at blocking droplets as regular surgical masks. However, they're effective enough to definitely be worthwhile if you don't have another option. The material you use matters, so we'll get into that in the next chapter.

While homemade masks aren't meant to protect healthy people from getting sick, it doesn't mean they are worthless. Any type of barrier between you and droplets must do something, right? A mask can also help prevent you from touching your nose and mouth. Wearing a mask isn't dangerous at all, so why not wear one as part of your safety protocol?

Pro: You can help the community

In times of crisis, medical supplies disappear fast. To help with the supply, you can make masks and find out where to donate them. Depending on the situation, the masks might not be used until absolutely necessary. A homemade mask is certainly better than a scarf or handkerchief. You can also make masks for your circle of friends and family who want them. This way, you won't contribute to the depletion of regular masks.

Con: Masks aren't effective if they aren't made properly

When you're buying a surgical mask, you know that it meets certain standards. When you make your own, however, it's up to you to make sure it's made properly. If you use the wrong material or it doesn't fit right, it basically becomes pointless. If you aren't familiar with sewing or crafting, the risk of making the mask incorrectly is higher. You want to be very careful when you're making your mask.

Con: Wearing a mask can give you a false sense of confidence

Let's be clear: wearing a mask if you aren't sick is only a potential win if you're doing other things to stay safe. This includes washing your hands properly (with soap and running water for at least 20 seconds), cleaning your environment, not touching your face, and avoiding direct contact with sick people if possible. Many people might wear a mask and feel that they're invincible. Unless the mask is an N95 respirator, it is not preventing you from inhaling particles, according to research. Even those masks are not very helpful if you aren't keeping up with good hygiene and disinfecting. This applies to sick people wearing masks, as well.

When should you wear your mask?

Here are some times when you should wear a mask:

- You are sick and want to protect the people taking care of you.

- You are taking care of someone who is sick and they need a mask.

- You are sick and need to go out to the store for groceries/supplies.

- You are sick and going to the doctor's office.

- You've been in contact with someone who is sick (you might be infected, but aren't showing symptoms yet).

- You are taking care of someone who is sick and want some kind of protection for yourself.

- You don't want people too close to you and wearing a mask might make people believe you are sick, so they'll give you a wide berth.

There is disagreement in the medical community about when to wear a mask. You might hear some experts say that even if you're healthy, you can wear a mask when you're in crowded areas and there's sickness going around. You'll also hear experts strongly proclaiming the opposite. This is most likely because they're worried about everyone buying masks. This will exhaust the supply for healthcare workers who really do need them. The fact that this is a debate is a big reason why it's a good idea to know how to make your own masks.

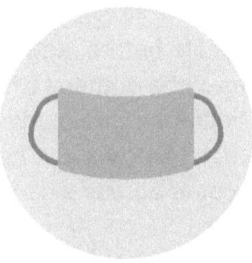

Chapter 3: Making a Mask

I hope you've read the first two chapters before this one. If not, that's okay, but just know that the previous chapters gave some important information on what masks can and can't do. I'm now going to talk about how to make your own surgical mask, which is designed to block droplets from sick people, therefore preventing the spread of disease. The mask isn't intended to protect you from getting sick. There are a handful of situations when experts recommend you wear one, though, like if you are healthy and caring for someone who is sick. There are also no risks to wearing a homemade mask (assuming you're also washing your hands, cleaning your environment, etc.), so we believe that if they make you feel safer, they're worth it.

N95 respirators, which *are* designed to protect healthy people from inhaling viruses, are made from very specific, specialized materials, so the vast majority of people can't make them by hand. Speaking of materials, that's the first topic we need to go over.

What materials work best for homemade masks?

You could make the best-looking mask ever, but if you used the wrong material, it won't be effective. Cambridge University performed a study of masks made from common household materials and how they compared to regular surgical masks. Vacuum cleaners bags performed the best, trapping 95% of droplet particles from a sick person. However, they were not easy to breathe through. Breathability is very important. If you can't breathe through your mask, you won't be able to wear it for very long. Not being able to breathe well is also dangerous for anyone with respiratory issues.

With breathability as a factor, the researchers concluded that cotton T-shirts, pillowcases, and anything else made from cotton were the best homemade mask materials. Cotton can trap about 50% of 0.2-micron particles.

I've never sewn anything before - what should I know?

If you haven't sewn anything in your life before, sewing a mask will probably be a bit challenging. It's a good idea to familiarize yourself with some basic terms and, if you know someone who does sew, ask them for help. Masks are still considered a good project for a beginner, though, so don't worry if you haven't been sewing a long time. Here are some of the terms you'll come across when starting to sew:

Seam - the line where you sew two pieces of fabric together

Seam allowance - the distance from the edge of the piece of cut fabric to the stitching

Clipping - you clip fabric by making snips in the seam allowance, but not into the stitching, so the fabric can open around curves or lay flat

Edgestitch - the line of stitching very close to a garment edge or seam line

Right side - the side of the fabric you want to be on the outside of your finished mask

Wrong side - the side of the fabric meant to be on the inside of the garment

Tuck - a fold or pleat in the fabric that's sewn into place

Straight stitch - a basic, straight stitched line

Topstitch - a line of stitching that's seen on the outside of the garment

Mask walkthrough

I recommend that you start with 100% cotton fabric. As we talked about before, cotton provides the best fabric in terms of protection and breathability. Here are the other supplies you'll need:

- Two 7-inch pieces of elastic

- Scissors

- Sewing supplies (needle and thread or sewing machine)

Important health note: Make sure the fabric you're using is clean. Washing it also makes it shrink a little, which will help with a tighter fit. You should also be sure to wash your hands before you get started.

1. If you're making a mask for an adult, cut out two 9x6-inch rectangles. For a child, the dimensions are 7.5x5-inches.

2. Line up the fabric rectangles, so you get two layers. Make sure the wrong side of the fabric is what's showing right now because eventually, you're turning the mask inside out. Put pins in the layers, so they don't shift as you sew.

3. If you haven't already, cut your elastic so each piece is 7-inches long.

If you want to make a pocket for a filter material, be sure to leave a small space (about 4-inches) on the long bottom side of the mask that isn't sewn closed. For filter materials, you have a few options, like spun-bound polypropylene. There are a handful of products that use this material, including frost cover fabric, waterproofing tape, weed covers, and mattress covers.

There's also cellulose polyester, which is a textile used for filtering gear oil, gasoline, and cleanroom wipes. Cleanroom wipes are used in "cleanrooms," which include areas like research labs and labs where medicines are made. Those are sensitive environments that need to be constantly monitored for airborne pollutants. The special cleanroom wipes could work as filters in your homemade mask.

People also use HEPA vacuum filters. Any filter you put in your mask still leaves gaps where the filter material isn't present. Because of this, it doesn't replace an N95, but if you can't access a respirator, a mask with a pocket filter is better than nothing.

4. Begin your sewing at the center of the bottom edge of your fabric rectangles. Sew to the first corner and stop, leaving a bit of space where the two parts aren't connected yet.

5. Now, you're going to sew the elastic with the edge out into the corner, so it is sewn between the two layers of the mask.

6. Turn your rectangle and sew to the next corner, making sure you aren't sewing on the elastic.

7. Move the other end of the elastic into the corner (it should be between the two layers of fabric still) and sew it with the edge in that corner.

8. Now for the top. Sew across the top to the next corner. Take your other piece of elastic, edge out in the corner, and sew.

9. Sew to the next corner and sew in the remaining end of your second piece of elastic.

10. Sew across the bottom, being sure to leave around 1.5-2 inches open. Cut the thread.

11. Turn the mask inside out. Pin three tucks on each side of the mask; this helps create a better fit. The tucks should be in the same direction.

12. The last step is to sew around the edge of the mask twice, so everything is as secure and tight as possible.

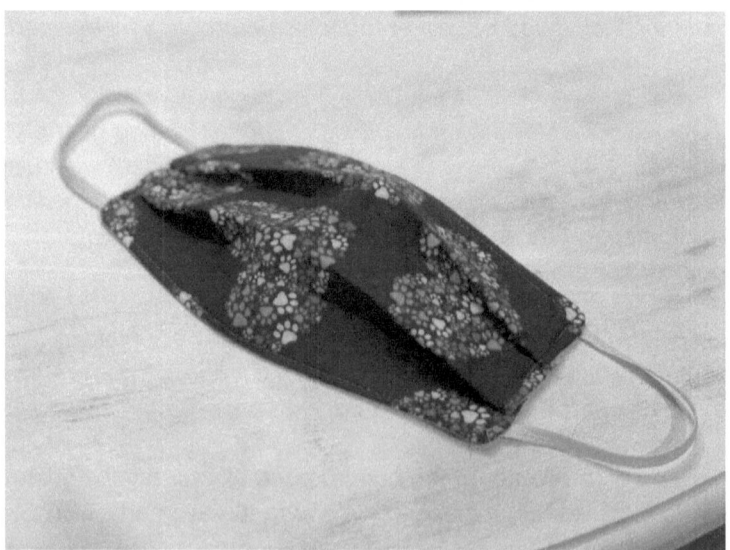

Can a homemade mask ever get close to a respirator?

There's been a little research on whether a homemade mask can replicate a real N95 respirator at all. In 2006, researchers did an experiment (Dato, Virginia M et al. "Simple respiratory mask." *Emerging infectious diseases* vol. 12,6 (2006): 1033-4) where they made a reusable cotton mask. They first boiled a Hanes Heavyweight 100% preshrunk cotton T-shirt for 10 minutes. After air-drying and sterilizing it, they cut out one outer layer and eight inner layers. They assembled it a specific way, so it wrapped around the wearer's head and covered their mouth and nose.

They then measured how well their homemade mask fit. They used an aerosol to see how well the mask worked at filtering out particles. While commercial N95 respirators have a fit of 100, the homemade mask fit one researcher at a 67. With larger faces, the fit reduced significantly. Overall, the researchers concluded that while their homemade mask did provide some protection and a decent fit, they could not advocate for its use as a substitute for a real respirator. There are a lot of factors at play like face size, variations in fabric material, and so on.

From this study, we can safely say that there hasn't been a good homemade version of a respirator. Regular surgical masks, yes, but not respirators. Remember that when making and using your homemade mask.

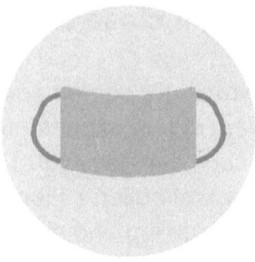

Chapter 4: How to Take Care of Your Mask

Once you've made a mask (or several masks), it's important to know how to handle and clean them properly. There's even a specific way you need to put on and remove the mask. In this chapter, I'll break down how to take care of your mask so it does its job protecting you.

How to put on and take off a mask

Before putting on your mask, wash your hands with soap and water. Make sure your mask is also clean before you put it on for the first time. If you can't remember if you've touched the inside of the mask or worry that someone else did, don't use it until it's been washed. If you know it's already clean, position the mask so it fits securely on your face. Once it's on, try not to mess with it. If you touch your mask while wearing it, wash your hands right away.

How long should you wear a mask?

You might be worried that a homemade mask could lose its effectiveness during use. In the same Cambridge University study that looked at mask material, they also looked at how the masks performed after 3 hours. Even with increased moisture and time, the masks essentially remained effective. However, experts recommend that you remove the mask as soon as it's damp.

Taking off the mask

Taking off the mask properly is very important. Both the front and inside of the mask are now contaminated. Grab the bottom and top elastic of the mask. Remove the mask without touching the front. Once it's removed, don't touch the inside of the mask. Wash your hands.

Washing your mask

Ideally, you want to wash the mask after each use. You *at least* want to wait to wear it again until after it's dry, but if you want to be as safe as possible, machine-wash after each use. To keep the mask in the best shape, choose a delicate setting. If you don't want to wait for the full washer/dryer time, you can boil a pot of water and hang the mask above it for 10 minutes. Air-dry before using again.

When to throw your mask away

Even handmade reusable masks shouldn't be used forever. As soon as you start to see damage, it's time to throw it away. Going through the washer and dryer a lot will break down the mask. Hand-washing your mask might help with its lifespan, but machine-washing on delicate is probably still a better way to go because it gives a much more thorough clean. If you feel your mask's fit getting looser, even after a wash, that's also a good sign that you need a new one.

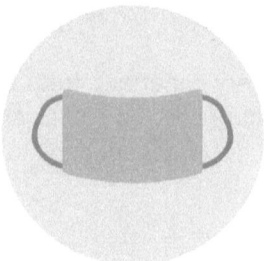

Chapter 5: Other Ways to Stay Safe from Microorganisms

As you've learned, wearing a mask is just one way to prevent the spread of disease. Other steps need to be taken or a mask can actually create a false sense of security. Whether you are sick or healthy, you need to do other things to keep you and others safe. In this chapter, I'll go through all the other ways to protect yourself from bacteria and viruses.

Wash your hands frequently and correctly

I can't overstate the importance of hand-washing. It's arguably the best defense humans have against sickness. Did you know that you can wash your hands the "wrong" way? Most people don't wash their hands enough and they don't wash them properly. Here are the times when you should wash your hands:

- Before you prepare food

- While you're preparing food (you touch raw meat, wash your hands before touching anything else)

- After you've prepared food

- Before you treat a wound

- After you treat a wound

- After you go to the bathroom

- After you change diapers

- After you clean up a child who used the bathroom

- After handling pet food

- After touching an animal, animal food, or animal waste

- After touching garbage

- Before you take care of someone who is sick

- After you take care of someone who is sick

Washing the right way

What's the right way to wash your hands? Rinse your hands with clean, running water. Put on the soap. Lather the soap, making sure to get all over your hands, including between your fingers, under your nails, and all the way up to your elbows. Scrub for at least 20 seconds. Rinse your hands in clean, running water. Dry with a clean towel or air-dry.

Using hand sanitizer

What if you don't have access to clean water and soap for some reason? You can also use a hand sanitizer. It needs to be at least 60% to be effective. Water and soap is still the best way to wash your hands, however, since hand sanitizers don't get rid of all kinds of germs. Hand sanitizers also don't work as well if your hands are clearly dirty or greasy. To use properly, squirt gel into your hands and rub all over until your hands feel completely dry.

Sanitize frequently-touched possessions and places in your home

Many microorganisms can survive for days on surfaces. You want to clean areas you touch a lot regularly. In your home, these areas include your kitchen and bathroom. To keep yourself safe, wear gloves while cleaning. First, wipe down areas with soap and water to get off grime and dust. Most EPA-registered cleaning products are sufficient.

To actually *sanitize,* you need something like a diluted bleach solution or disinfectant wipe. When using diluted household bleach, make sure it works for the surface you're cleaning. You also want to make sure you aren't exposing yourself to fumes, so work with windows open. You should never mix bleach with other cleaners. Dilute with water.

What else do you touch a lot?

Once you've cleaned your bathroom and kitchen, think about other areas that you touch a lot. This includes door handles and light switches. It also includes electronics. Most people would be horrified at how many germs live on their cell phones. Cleaning electronics is a little tricky because you can't just use soap and water. Even hand sanitizer sprays aren't great. Luckily, you can find electronic-specific sanitizer wipes that can be used on phones, TV screens, remotes, and more. Different brands will offer recommendations as well. As an example, Apple says you can use Clorox disinfectant wipes.

If you don't have these wipes around and are concerned about germs, you can *very carefully* use a clean microfiber cloth and rubbing alcohol. Never apply your cleaner directly to the phone or screen; always apply it to the cloth. The cloth should be just slightly damp. You'll see different ideas around the internet like diluted vinegar, but there will always be another source saying not to do it. If you're using anything that isn't a commercially-made electronics wipe, be very careful. Don't forget to clean phone and laptop cases, too!

How often do you need to clean?

In a perfect world, you would be cleaning a little every day, but that's not something most people will do. To keep yourself safe, at least once a week should be okay. If someone in the house is sick, however, you do want to commit to cleaning every day.

Keep up with laundry

Germs can survive on clothes and towels. If people share clothing, towels, or blankets, they can spread germs to one another. Touching dirty laundry with your hand can also get germs on your hands. Getting sick from dirty laundry is more likely if you've been caring for someone who is sick and you get their bodily fluids on your clothes. According to the Cleveland Clinic, you want to be sure to wash "high-risk" items sooner rather than later in hot water with a bleach-based cleaning product. High-risk items include soiled clothes, athletic clothes, healthcare worker uniforms, and so on. If someone in your home has an infectious disease, you want to keep up with laundry to prevent spreading.

Get vaccinated

Health organizations like the WHO and CDC recommend vaccinations as one of the best ways to protect yourself from diseases. Vaccinations not only protect individuals, but they also contribute to herd immunity and help reduce disease in those who aren't immunized. Vaccine-preventable diseases include diphtheria, hepatitis B, measles, meningitis, mumps, rubella, tuberculosis, and yellow fever. Seasonal flu vaccines are also produced and offered to the public. To reduce your chances of getting sick and protect your community, keep up on your recommended vaccinations.

Cover your mouth when you sneeze or cough

Many diseases spread by droplets. To protect the people around you, always cover your mouth and nose when you sneeze or cough. If you can, use a tissue to catch your cough or sneeze. If that's not an option, cover your mouth and nose with the inside of your elbow. This prevents the spray of germs from getting into the air.

Don't touch your face

Microorganisms get into your body through places like your nose, mouth, and eyes. Even if you're washing your hands frequently, you can easily pick something up during the day. When you touch your face (rubbing your eyes, chewing your nails, etc.), you can infect yourself. Avoid touching your face. Wearing a mask can help you remember if you're really concerned about what you might put in your body.

Stay at home if you're sick

If you're feeling sick, stay at home until you're well again. Educate yourself on your employer's rules about sick leave and days off. Know what your city/state's laws on sick leave are, too. I realize that taking time off from work may be an issue for some people, especially hourly workers. It's something that each person will have to decide for themselves, but if you are sick, do be aware that coming into work anyway puts others at risk. While your symptoms may not be too bad, the germs you carry could be devastating for someone else.

Practice social distancing

When there's an illness going around, keep distance between you and others. If you see someone coughing, sneezing, or displaying other symptoms, give them a wide berth. The germs they spray into the air can survive there for a while. If you're too close, you can breathe them in. If you are the one that's sick, follow proper social distancing courtesy. If possible, stay at home. Wear a mask if you have to go out somewhere. Don't go to areas where you know lots of people might gather or hug/kiss your loved ones.

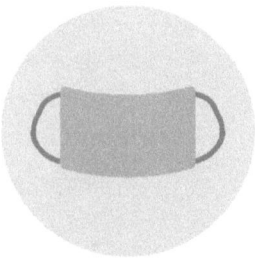

Conclusion

Homemade masks, when made and used properly, play an important part in slowing the spread of disease. Studies show that household materials like 100% cotton get close to surgical masks in terms of effectiveness. Remember, that's when the person who is sick wears the mask. Homemade masks don't prevent you from inhaling virus particles. Homemade masks can be used when you're caring for someone who is sick and when you need a reminder to not touch your face. In times of crisis, many hospitals and clinics will put out calls for homemade masks, as well.

This book taught you how to make your own mask and how to care for it. I hope the book was useful to you and that you now have an understanding of when and why to use masks. They are just a part of safety precautions that can keep you, your family, and your community protected from disease. Wash your hands, don't touch your face, stay home when you're sick, and practice social distancing when necessary. Disease is scary, but if we're all careful and educate ourselves, we can make a positive difference in our world.